Eliminate Your Headaches in Less Than 30 Days

A Holistic Approach

Dr. John M. Anderson

© 2014 by Dr. John M. Anderson

ISBN-10: 099605362X
ISBN-13: 978-0-9960536-2-4

All Rights Reserved. No part of this publication may be reproduced in any form or by any means, including scanning, photocopying, or otherwise without prior written permission of the copyright holder.

First Printing, 2014

Printed in the United States of America

Liability Disclaimer

The author of this book does not dispense medical advice or prescribe the use of any technique as a form of treatment for physical or medical problems without the advice of a physician, either directly or indirectly. The intent of the author is only to offer information of a general nature to help you in your quest for health and well-being. In the event you use any of the information in this book for yourself, which is your constitutional right, the author assumes no responsibility for your actions.

Eliminate Your Headaches in Less Than 30 Days

A Holistic Approach

Table of Contents

Introduction -- 9

Why Headaches and Neck Pain Are So Common Today ------ 15

Types of Headaches & Their Symptoms -------------------------- 19

Common Symptoms (The Common Denominators) ----------- 25

The Typical Treatment Plan & Why It Doesn't Work --------- 39

The Holistic Approach to Eliminating Your Headaches in Less Than 30 Days -- 49

Diet for Headache Relief: A Precautionary Measure ---------- 65

Personal Case Studies -- 79

FAQ's -- 89

APPENDIX A -- 95

Introduction

Are headaches ruining your life? Do you miss work due to headaches or migraines? Do headaches affect your ability to enjoy life to the fullest? If you answered yes to any of the above questions, you are not alone.

According to the National Headache Foundation, over 45 million people suffer from chronic recurring headaches, and of the 28 million who suffer from migraines, about 20% are children and adolescents.

Many years ago while studying martial arts, I was allowing myself to be put in a headlock during a training demonstration when I felt a sharp pull on the right side of my neck. Afterward, I felt fine, nothing that a little Advil couldn't help, so I continued my martial arts training and completely forgot about the incident.

About a year later, I noticed that I was starting to get one or two headaches per week, usually originating from the right side of my neck. This was something that I had never experienced in the past. Over the next couple of years, the headaches got more and more frequent, about four to five per week, and I noticed I was relying on medication to get through the day.

In looking at the cause of headaches and doing some post graduate studies, I found that most headaches today, including migraines, are really muscle tension headaches. These headaches have a musculo-skeletal component, which means that any past injury, such as auto accidents, even minor fender benders that most people overlook, can be a major contributing factor. I had overlooked what I thought was a minor martial arts injury, but what I realized is that it had set me up for a chronic headache syndrome that started a year later.

Now, as a chiropractor, I should have known better, but up until that time, my practice consisted mainly of treating lower back pain. In the 1980's and 1990's, most chiropractic research was done on lower back pain syndrome and all of the studies showed very favorable results.

Initially, my research began by evaluating my diet. I found that certain foods seemed to contribute to my headaches and that caffeine seemed to eliminate my headaches. Although I loved to eat cheese on crackers, I found that certain cheeses, such as aged cheese, seemed to give rise to a headache. Red wine was another culprit. Of course, aged cheese and red wine seemed to go really well together! In doing further research, I found that certain foods, including nitrates and some food colorings, increase blood flow to the brain, causing headaches in some people.

Something else my research led to has to do with body positioning and sleep ergonomics. I found that if I took a nap on the sofa or fell asleep watching TV with pillows under my head, I usually woke up with a stiff neck and would get a headache within the next 24 hours.

Stress was another offender, especially mental stress. I noticed that if I had a particularly stressful situation at work or home, even though I thought the problem was resolved, I usually woke up the next morning with a stiff neck and a resultant headache.

I realized that I needed to address all of these issues if I was going to get a handle on my headaches. Over 45 million Americans each year, one out of every six, suffer from chronic headaches. In this book, I will explain why that is. I'll explain what the "typical" treatment plan is and why it doesn't address the problem. Then, I'll present an effective, common sense approach to dramatically reduce, if not totally eliminate, your headaches within the next 30 days.

Why Headaches and Neck Pain Are So Common Today

Today, neck pain and headaches are extremely common for adults, children and senior citizens alike. There are, of course, a small percentage of people whose headaches may be a result of a severe disease process. The majority of people, however, can be helped through a common sense approach, because most headaches are a result of the typical American diet, bad posture and past injuries.

Certain foods can elicit or set up headaches. Stress, both physical and emotional, can also have a direct effect on the "fight or flight" mechanism, stimulating an increase in adrenaline flow, which causes an elevation of blood pressure.

In today's society, the use of computers has quadrupled over the last 10 years. The problem is not the computer, but the ergonomic position it puts us in. Typically, while spending more than 30 minutes on a laptop or desktop computer, most of us tend lean forward, putting the head in a forward position over the shoulders, causing stress and tension in the muscles of the neck and upper back area. This posture is commonly known as Forward Head Posture (FHP), and it generally happens when the computer screen is too low, coupled with the repetitive motion of moving the head forward to read the screen. This position causes tension and stress on the neck and sub-occipital muscles.

Unfortunately, FHP isn't limited to adults. The over-use of video games, texting and computer use have begun to affect many at a very young age. Most teen and preteen children spend hours sitting in one position, causing the body to adapt to this bad posture. As a result, it's not uncommon for preteen children to experience headaches and neck pain.

Types of Headaches & Their Symptoms

There are many different types of primary headaches. Although all headaches are different, they all have at least one thing in common – they cause pain.

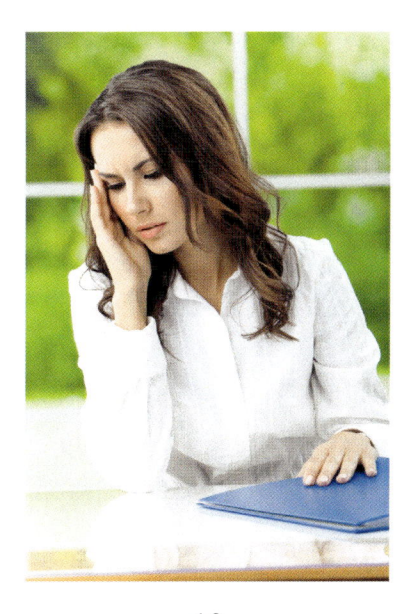

Let's look at the different types now:

Episodic Tension Headaches (the most common form of headache)

- Occur less than 15 days per month
- Mild to moderate pain
- Constant band-like pain, pressure or throbbing
- Affects the front, top or sides of the head
- May last from 30 minutes to several days
- Usually brought on by neck tension, stress, poor diet, certain foods, lack of food or preservatives

Chronic Tension Headaches

- Occur more than 15 days per month
- Varying intensity pain throughout the day, but it is almost always present

- Affects the front, top or sides of the head

- Pain comes and goes over a prolonged time period

- Usually associated with chronic cervical subluxation, forward head posture (FHP), and long-term dietary issues like food allergies (gluten, tyramine, MSG, aspartame, nitrates or nitrites)

- Symptoms may include: a headache upon awakening, difficulty falling asleep and staying asleep, irritability, disturbed concentration, mild sensitivity to light or nausea, and general muscle aching

Migraines

- Can occur in various combinations and include moderate to severe pain, often described as pounding or throbbing

- Can affect the whole head or can shift from one side of the head to another

- Symptoms may include: sensitivity to light, noise or odors, blurred vision, nausea, vomiting and upset stomach, abdominal pain, loss of appetite, sensations of being very warm or very cold, paleness, fatigue, dizziness, bright flashing dots of light, blind spots, or an aura of wavy or jagged lines

Cluster Headaches

- Intense one-sided pain described as having a burning or piercing quality that is throbbing or constant

- Pain is located in one eye or in one eye region without changing sides

- Pain generally lasts 30-90 minutes, but can extend to three or four hours

- These headaches come and go throughout the day (most sufferers get 1-3 headaches per day during a cluster period)

Sinus Headaches

- Deep and constant pain in the cheekbones, forehead or bridge of the nose

- Pain usually intensifies with sudden head movement or straining

- Usually occurs with other sinus symptoms, such as nasal discharge, feeling of fullness in the ears, fever and facial swelling

Common Symptoms (The Common Denominators)

Since muscle tension headaches are by far the most common, let's talk about them first. Most tension headaches take time to develop and can be brought on or exacerbated by physical or emotional stress. This type of headache is often misdiagnosed as a migraine and can vary in severity. Muscles tension headache can last from a few hours to days in more severe cases.

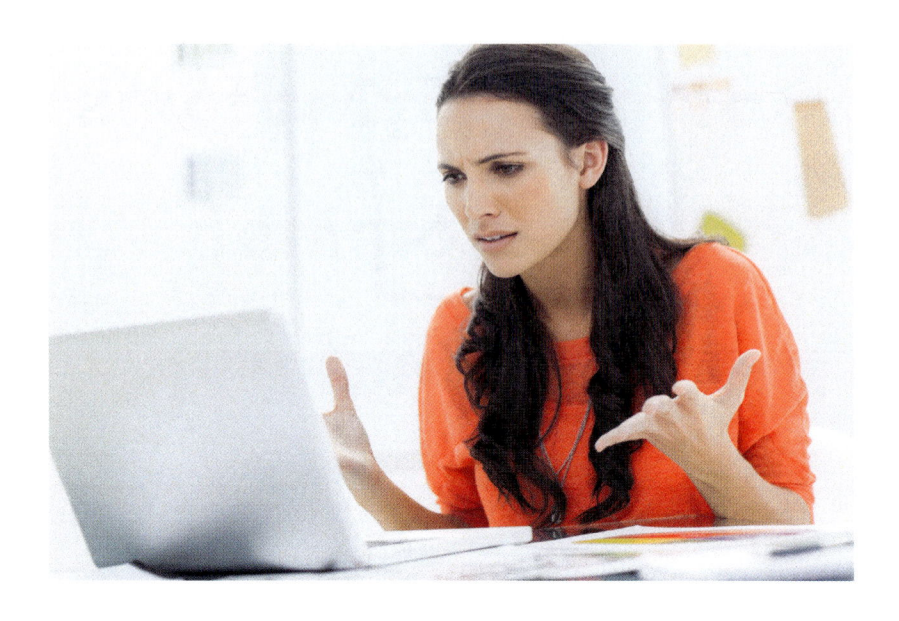

This type of headache tends to form as a result of muscle contraction. It's commonly felt as a band behind the eyes, and often is more focused on one side than the other. Sometimes patients complain of tension at the base of the skull, which radiates through the head into the back of the eyes. If the headache persists more than a couple of hours, nausea and sensitivity to light and sound can commonly accompany the progression of symptoms. This type of headache can be and is usually recurrent if the tension or stress is not relieved.

Most specialists today are realizing that if left untreated, many tension headaches can turn into the classic migraine. Recently, doctors have come up with a new term called the "mixed tension migraine," which has characteristics of both a tension headache and a migraine headache.

Medical professionals believe that migraines are caused by changes in the blood flow to the brain. Millions of people worldwide experience regular migraine headaches.[i] Tension headaches, which are caused by muscle stress and tension, are even more common. According to the World Health Organization, this headache type affects over 70 percent of some populations.[ii]

According to Harvard Health, scientists believe that a continuum of headaches exist, with tension headaches at one end and migraines at the other.[iii] Since mixed tension migraines have symptoms of both migraines and tension headaches, they are thought to be somewhere in the middle of the headache continuum. In both muscle tension headaches and diagnosed migraine headaches, intracranial blood vessel dilation (expanding) seems to be a common denominator.

Usually, a person that is suffering from a muscle contraction, tension-type headache will also have symptoms of neck pain or stiffness. In doing a case history, I found that some of the more common causes of this type of headache include:

1. A career in which the person's head is brought into a forward head posture, making him or her spend a predominant part of the day looking down or forward, i.e. working on a computer, desk work, writing, charting or even machine shop or factory work.

2. Past motor vehicle accidents, even minor ones, past sports injuries and falls. Many of these can have taken place many years before, and can later have an effect on the segmental alignment of the vertebrae. These past injuries can easily be overlooked, but can frequently show up as a recurring problem many years later.

According to Dr. I. A. Kapandji, M.D, author of *Physiology of the Joints, Volume 3*, "for every inch of Forward Head Posture, it can increase the weight of the head on the spine by an additional 10 pounds."[iv]

Couple that with the fact that when your head is in a forward position, a facet joint separation and spinal instability is caused, and you can understand the increasing amount of muscle tension and stress in these areas. As you can see, over time, the amount of tension that is continually placed on the muscle supporting the weight of the head can have detrimental effects.

Sleeping is another potential problem, especially when there are too many pillows involved. Sleeping on the couch while watching TV is a common practice that puts the head in a forward position, which can assist in losing the natural curvature of the neck.

Why is a loss of natural cervical curvature and avoiding forward head posture so important? When there is a normal cervical curvature (cervical lordosis), there is very little tension on the muscles of the neck and upper back since the top cervical vertebrae lines up in a perpendicular line with the bottom vertebrae.

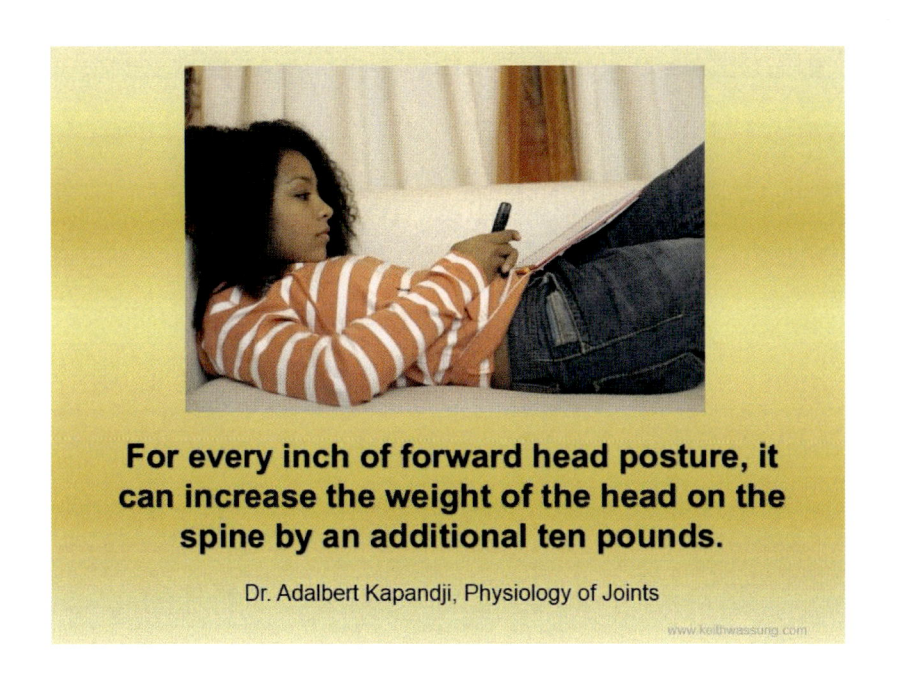

For every inch of forward head posture, it can increase the weight of the head on the spine by an additional ten pounds.

Dr. Adalbert Kapandji, Physiology of Joints

The joints that support the spinal column are called facet joints. They carry the weight and add stability to the entire spine. When one has a loss of the normal cervical curvature, facet joint separation is the result. This separation of the facet joints will cause an instability and lack of support to the spine. The body's natural response is to contract (tighten) the muscle, therefore trying to add stability – this is what the Autonomic Nervous System does to protect your central nervous system (brain and spinal cord). This tightening of the muscles is called muscle guarding or muscle splinting, but most people refer to it as a muscle spasm. There is always a cause and effect—the <u>cause</u> being Forward Head Posture (facet separation) and the <u>effect</u> being tight, achy muscles that often turn into a muscle tension or migraine headache.

Many headaches originate from the upper cervical spine and can be felt on palpation as acute trigger points at C1-C2 on the lateral side of the neck on an initial exam. Just because a person has a misalignment (subluxation) at C1-C2 and a forward head posture doesn't always mean it will dramatically effect or reduce a person's range of motion. Not surprisingly, because of muscle compensation, although you may be suffering from muscle tension headaches, you may have a mostly normal range of motion and many times negative orthopedic testing.

The standard American diet, especially processed foods, is another common denominator that can have a direct effect on a person's susceptibility to headaches and muscle tension. High carbohydrate diets can also be a major player. Arteries are affected by insulin, and most cells in the body need to burn glucose with oxygen to produce energy. The digestive system breaks down carbohydrates, helping the glucose to migrate from the blood into the cells. The pancreas responds with a strong hit of insulin, and this sudden drop in blood sugar seems to encourage the arteries in the head to constrict, leading to a rebound effect due to a lack of blood flow and oxygen. In order to compensate, the body's self protective mechanism causes an increase in vasodilatation, therefore increasing intracranial blood pressure and inducing a headache. Skipping medication can also cause a drop in sugar levels and is another common factor with people who have insulin-related headaches.

What Actually Causes a Headache, Medically Speaking

For those of you who want a little more information about what actually takes place inside your body when you are having a headache, this section is for you. I kept it short and sweet to provide only as much info as is necessary to give you a more complete understanding of your body and your headaches. Once you realize what is actually happening, you will gain a more comprehensive understanding of what causes and what might prevent your headaches. There are five parts of the body that are affected when a headache is taking place:

The Meninges

The meninges is the tissue that holds your brain in place and keeps it from knocking against your skull. The dura mater has a lot of blood vessels running through it and is very sensitive to pain. The dura extends into the spinal canal and protects the spinal cord. Any twisting or torsion of the dura shows up as a headache.

Blood Supply

The brain and meninges are supplied with blood from arteries from the internal carotid, vertebral basilar and external carotid arteries. Meningal blood vessels are very sensitive to pain, and it is generally accepted that the development of headaches depends upon irritation of these sensitive nerves.

Trigeminal Nerve

Dilated meningal blood vessels send pain signals via a branch of the trigeminal nerve. These nerves then signal to the thalamus and higher brain centers where they are perceived as pain. This is known as the trigeminal autonomic reflex.

Facial Nerve

Similar to the trigeminal nerve, the facial nerve has synapses in the cervical region of the spine, also sending signals to higher brain centers where they are perceived as pain.

Cerebral Spinal Fluid

The CSF is made in your brain, travels through your sinus, is protected by the dura mater throughout the spine, and then comes back into the brain.

In each of the above causes of headaches there is one common denominator: the neck. This is because a subluxation, or misalignment, of the top vertebra of the neck can:

1. Cause tension and torsion of the meninges

2. Cause changes in the blood pressure and size of blood vessels in the head
3. Interfere with nerve input and output of the trigeminal nerve
4. Impair normal CSF flow throughout the cranium and spine

It should be noted that there are two basic types of headaches: primary headaches, which we described above, and secondary headaches, which are secondary to disease process. A thorough evaluation should always be done before classification or treatment begins.

Next, we'll talk about the typical treatment plan, why it doesn't usually work, and finally, a real life "common sense solution" to reduce or totally eliminate your headaches in the next 30 days.

The Typical Treatment Plan & Why It Doesn't Work

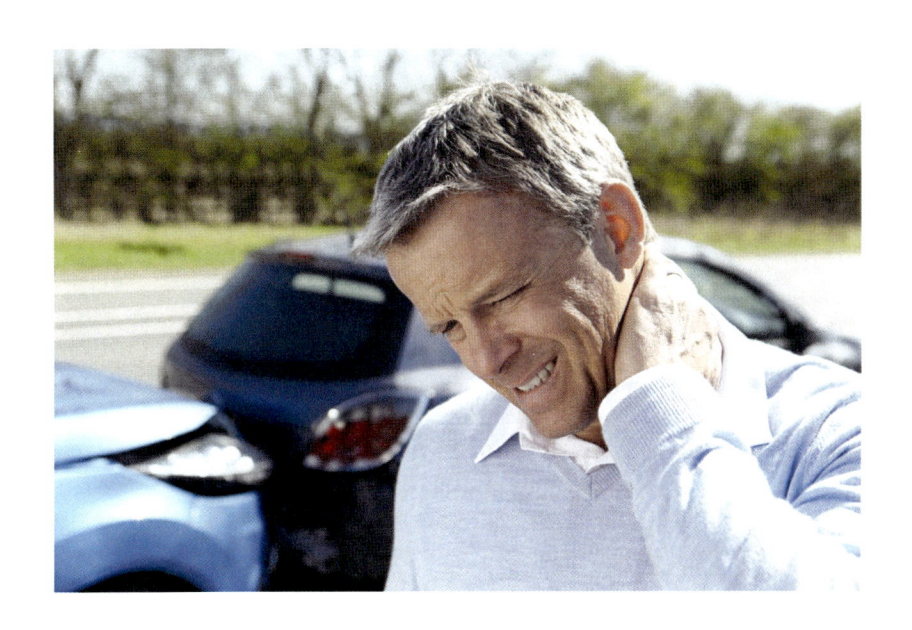

Many times, when a person is suffering from neck pain or a headache, the first thing on their mind is obviously to get out of pain. Typically, most people will just reach for Tylenol (acetaminophen), Motrin or Advil (ibuprofen), or Aleve (naproxen sodium). Although these over-the-counter medications may offer temporary relief, there is a risk of becoming reliant on them in order to get through the week. Many people make the mistake of using these drugs as a permanent solution to the problem.

If you've watched any commercials for these drugs, you know they give off the impression that daily, regular use of these medications will lead to a happier, pain free life. What the commercials won't tell you, however, is that the chronic side effects of these drugs can be damaging to your health and sometimes even fatal. Unfortunately, this is so common in our society, that the drug companies amass millions of dollars each year in clever marketing to trick the consumer.

Let's look at the facts associated with acetaminophen, the top brand being Tylenol. Acetaminophen, also called paracetamol, is not a NSAID (non-steroidal anti-inflammatory drug), but a distinct analgesic and fever-reducing drug with a similar brand usage.[v]

An acetaminophen overdose is the leading cause of acute liver failure in the developed world, accounting for more than 56,000 emergency room visits, 26,000 hospitalizations and 450 deaths per year in the U.S. Acetaminophen can also contribute to kidney toxicity.[vi]

Although the "safe" dose of acetaminophen is up to 4 grams per day, chronic daily ingestion of this dose has been shown to cause elevations of liver enzymes, even in healthy people, which indicates liver irritation and inflammation, which can lead to permanent liver damage. Furthermore, since alcohol, especially when consumed chronically, increases the toxic potential of acetaminophen, many people unknowingly put themselves at risk of serious liver damage by consuming acetaminophen and alcohol together.[vii]

Acetaminophen has been available as an over-the-counter drug for over 50 years. More than 100 million people use acetaminophen in the U.S. alone, with up to 50 million Americans using acetaminophen-containing products in a given week.[viii] Acetaminophen accounts for up to 50 percent of all adult cases of acute liver failure in the U. S. Even in the absence of overt overdose symptoms, therapeutic acetaminophen dosages can still increase concentrations of liver enzymes, which are markers of liver damage.[ix]

Other potential negative consequences of acetaminophen include increased risk of fracture, inhibition of testosterone production, and kidney toxicity.

As you can see, regular usage of Tylenol (acetaminophen) to treat chronic neck pain, headaches or anything else may not be such a good idea.

Other drugs commonly used for headache relief are a group called NSAiDs (non-steroidal anti inflammatory drugs), which include ibuprofen (Motrin and Advil), aspirin and naproxen (Aleve). In contrast to the liver toxicity of acetaminophen, NSAiDs exhibit varying degrees of gastrointestinal, cardiovascular and kidney toxicity. NSAiDs, such as aspirin and ibuprofen, are Cox1 and Cox2 inhibitors. Inhibition of Cox1 results in degradation of the protective mucous layer of the stomach. Damage to the lining of the stomach and small intestine results in symptoms that range from relatively minor heartburn, nausea and abdominal pain (affecting 15-40% of

NSAiD users) to life-threatening ulceration, perforation and bleeding (affecting 1-2% of chronic NSAiD users).[x]

Further, NSAiDs can lead to Cox2 inhibition, causing blood vessel constriction, which can increase the risk of thrombosis and heart attack as well as hypertension, kidney toxicity and renal failure. For more technical information on the affect of NSAiDs on Cox 1 and Cox 2, see Appendix A.[xi]

In a study involving more than 10,000 elderly individuals, long-term, high-dose NSAiD therapy was associated with a significant risk of progression of chronic kidney disease. Sometimes, irregularities in kidney function are even observed in NSAiD users with healthy kidneys. Other consequences of kidney toxicity related to NSAiD use include high blood pressure, salt and water retention, and electrolyte imbalances.

As noted by Life Extension's article called *Acetaminophen and NSAID Toxicity*[xii], here are several factors that influence the risk of toxicity of NSAiD use:

- **Age** – Individuals over 60 years old are 5-6 times more likely to develop NSAiD-related ulcers.
- **Medical Conditions** – Prior history of gastrointestinal complications increases the risk of NSAiD ulcers by 4-5 times. Cardiovascular or respiratory disease, renal or hepatic impairment, diabetes, rheumatoid arthritis and hypertension are also accounted with increased risk.
- **Dose and Duration** – The use of high dose NSAiDs increases the risk of gastrointestinal complications up to tenfold, while duration of use appears to increase the risk of cardiovascular problems.

Medical intervention is always a better choice than self-medication. For short-term relief, it is always safer to be under medical care. Triptans are usually the first prescription of choice, but are not without their side effects. They function by constricting or narrowing the blood vessels in order to keep chemicals that are thought to cause migraines from being released.

When triptans are taken often, however, they can cause rebound headaches, which are headaches that are caused by taking too much medication. Other side effects are nausea and dizziness, muscle weakness and abnormal heart rhythms. Although these medications work for treating the symptoms of many people and are always helpful in an emergency situation, they are not long-term solutions.

My goal for this book is to help people become less reliant on medication and to focus on the cause and prevention of neck pain and headaches by improving posture and changing diet to improve overall health.

The Holistic Approach to Eliminating Your Headaches in Less Than 30 Days

As I've demonstrated, treating headaches and migraines the traditional way is not the answer. It simply covers up the real problem and wreaks havoc on other areas of your health in the meantime. The only way to live headache-free is to make some lifestyle changes that result in a healthier way of being. The holistic approach to eliminating headaches that I am suggesting is one that will improve your overall health, allowing you to live from a state of wellness that is not conducive to headaches.

The changes that I am asking you to make are not difficult when you consider what you have been dealing with. If you are reading this book, it is likely that your headaches have been affecting your life so much that you'll do just about anything to make them stop. Remember that as you go through this section because there will likely be times when it seems easier to just pop a pill. These steps have the power to transform your life into one that is headache-free! This approach puts you in the driver's seat of your own health, and that is where you want to be.

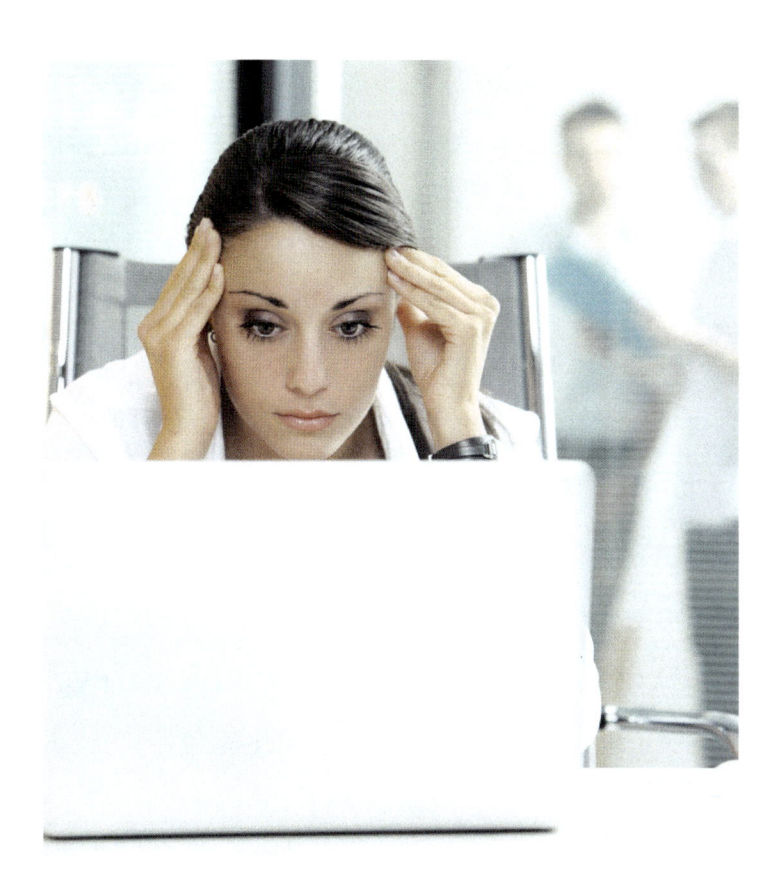

Step 1: Diagnose Your Headache Type

Do you know what type of headaches you suffer from? Are they tension headaches? Are they migraines? Or are they another type altogether? There are many different types of headaches. Before an appropriate treatment plan can be laid out, proper diagnosis is most important so that you can determine the type of headache you are suffering from.

Although all signs and symptoms point to a muscle tension headache, an MRI of the brain and cervical spine can be performed to rule out any other primary cause. Then, an anterior to posterior open-mouth x-ray of the cervical spine with a lateral cervical spine is performed to evaluate spinal alignment. A common misalignment (subluxation) seen on the A-P view is a C1-C2 rotation. Misalignment of the top two cervical vertebrae can affect vertebral artery flow and is a very common condition with people who suffer from muscle tension headaches.

Another common condition seen on the x-ray of the lateral cervical spine is a loss of the cervical curve (loss of lordosis), which can cause facet joint separation and muscle tension in the back of the neck, and can then continue into the upper shoulder and mid-back area.

Step 2: Correct Forward Head Posture

One way of correcting Forward Head Posture is by using a specific type of traction called a Lordotic Cervical Traction Pump. By using an air-pressure gauge similar to a blood pressure pump, each individual can control the amount of force applied to the traction. There is a gradual increase in force applied, which is measured by the number of pumps over a 30 day period used 15-20 minutes per day. The goal is to help reduce tension in the muscles of the cervical spine by reducing the cervical kyphosis (general bad posture). After 30 days, continued treatment is recommended at home for two times a week to help maintain proper cervical lordosis. This is especially true if you have a long history of muscle tension headaches, and post motor vehicle accidents. If you have a computer-oriented career, you will also find this helpful in maintaining proper posture and reducing muscle tension, and it is also effective as a preventative measure.

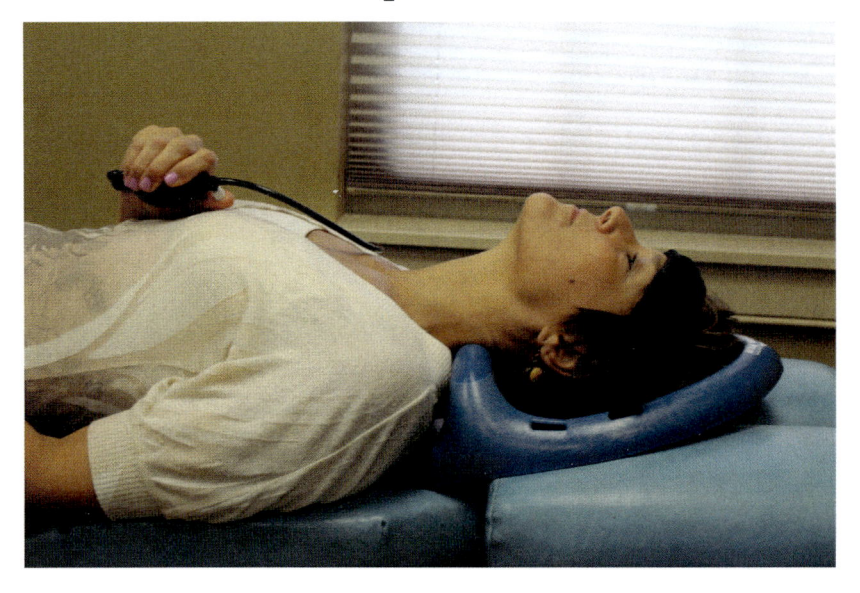

Patient using a lordotic cervical traction pump

Step 3: Evaluate Trigger Points

Another part of treatment for muscle tension headaches is to evaluate the muscles individually that are the main source of the trigger points. Evaluating each muscle is primarily done with a very careful and specific muscle palpation to document precisely what muscles are active (very tender). Trigger points usually are our body's way of protecting us from more severe damage. Misalignment of the vertebrae of the cervical spine can cause nerve pressure, spinal cord pressure and constriction of blood vessels that flow through the vertebral arteries. Our body's way of protecting us and compensating is to tighten up certain muscles to add stability. This is called muscle guarding or muscle splinting, but most people refer to it as a muscle spasm.

Trigger points need to be addressed, specifically with deep tissue work and myofascial release techniques, to elongate the muscle belly, reduce muscle contractions and restore normal movement of the muscle. Myofascial release techniques, along with chiropractic adjustments that correct the misaligned vertebrae and lordotic cervical traction, are the keys to restoring normal segmental motion and to bringing the supportive muscles back to a stabilized and balanced position. Once this is accomplished after 30 days of treatment, a series of home stretching exercises, along with lordotic cervical traction needs to be done on a bi-weekly basis. The lordotic cervical traction is accomplished by a device called a Posture Pump. Neck Stretches should be done on a daily basis.

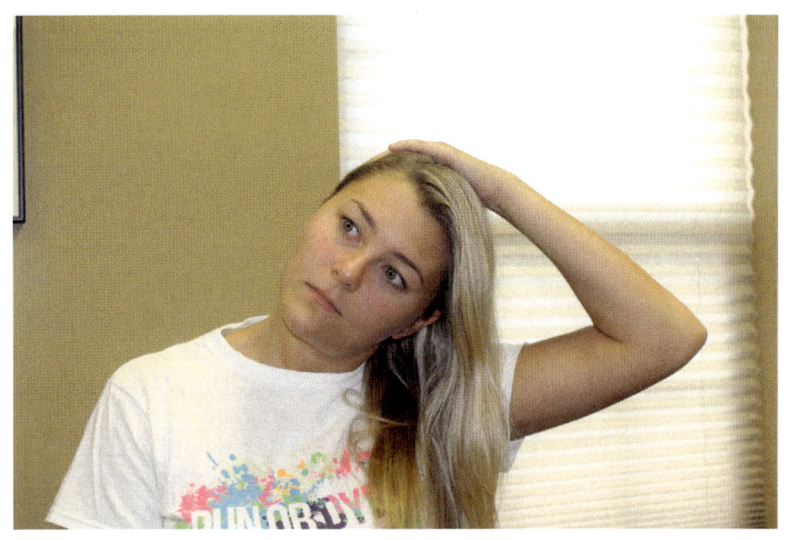

Patient doing lateral neck stretch

Step 4: Make Ergonomic Changes

The following ergonomic corrective changes and habits are important to make since they will help you maintain a posture that reduces the risk of headaches:

- Eliminate all forward head posture positions in order for corrective changes to be able to reduce and last. Move your desk components, computer equipment and devices into a placement that helps you eliminate forward head posture. Avoid prolonged texting and elevate all computers to eye level.
- Use a lumbar support in the lower back to stabilize the upper cervical spine (both the lumbar and cervical spine has lordotic curves).

- Sleep with only one pillow, preferably a memory foam pillow with a cervical curve built in.
- Avoid reading in bed or falling asleep while watching TV. Habits like these that put your head in a forward head position will only aggravate the condition and ensure the chance of recurring tension headaches.

Step 5: Eat a Diet That Reduces the Risk of Headaches

Another major factor to be considered in the treatment of headaches is the evaluation of a person's diet. Certain foods have been known to cause or initiate a headache, especially if an individual has an ergonomic predisposition like forward head posture. Foods that are high in tyramine, such as processed meats, pickles, onions, olives, and canned soups, along with aged cheese and red wine are among these foods. Other common chemicals that have been shown to have an effect on the arteries of the heart and therefore can cause headaches include monosodium glutamate (MSG), a common flavor enhancer that is often simply listed as "natural flavorings" on the ingredients label. Nitrates, generally found in processed meats, are another stimulator of headaches.

Food colorings, aspartame, preservatives and other additives are also notorious for promoting headaches and triggering migraines. These should also be eliminated from your diet, especially as they serve no nutritional value at all.

By eliminating the above foods or even reducing their intake, you will be taking a big step in the right direction. This, alone, will have a profound effect in reducing the frequency and intensity of headaches. Diet is so important when it comes to stopping headaches, however, that I've dedicated the entire next chapter to it.

Step 6: Exercise More Consistently

Engaging in exercises that reduce stress is another important method for reducing headaches. You might consider taking up walking, swimming or especially yoga.

Here is what the Mayo clinic has to say about yoga specifically:

"Yoga is a mind–body practice that combines stretching exercises, controlled breathing, and relaxation. Yoga can help reduce stress, lower blood pressure and improve heart function. And almost anyone can do it. Yoga is considered a mind-body complementary and alternative medicine practice. Yoga brings together physical and mental disciplines to achieve peacefulness of body and mind, helping you relax and manage stress and anxiety.

Yoga has many styles, forms and intensities. Hatha yoga, in particular, may be a good choice for stress management. Hatha is one of the most common styles of yoga, and beginners may like its slower pace and easier movements. But most people can benefit from any style of yoga; it is all about your personal preferences."[xiii]

In summary, poor cervical spine posture, and forward head posture, can be reduced by:

1. <u>Proper ergonomic changes</u> or avoiding a forward head position at home and at work.
2. <u>Chiropractic adjustments</u> to correct subluxation caused by past motor vehicle accidents, sports injuries, falls and bad posture.
3. <u>Myofascial release techniques</u> to reduce trigger points brought on by muscle guarding.

Usually within 30 days of active treatment, defined as three times per week, there is substantial improvement and a reduction in the frequency and intensity of neck pain and headaches. Since about 90 percent of all headaches are muscle tension or mixed tension headaches (muscle contraction/migraine), this type of treatment will be helpful in reducing or eliminating most headaches.

Diet for Headache Relief: A Precautionary Measure

Quite a few people have shown positive results in reducing headaches on the Paleo Diet, which can be summarized as "any food eaten without being processed." In this case, processed foods include not only packaged foods, but also grains, bread, pasta and pasteurized dairy. What is recommended is lots of fresh fruit and vegetables, nuts and oils, along with organic poultry, grass fed lean meats and wild caught fish. Organic eggs can be eaten as well. The following websites contain helpful information on healthy eating and the Paleo Diet:

1. Local Harvest: http://localharvestgrocery.com
2. USDA Farmers Market Listing: http://search.ams.usda.gov/farmersmarkets
3. Eat Wild: http://www.eatwild.com

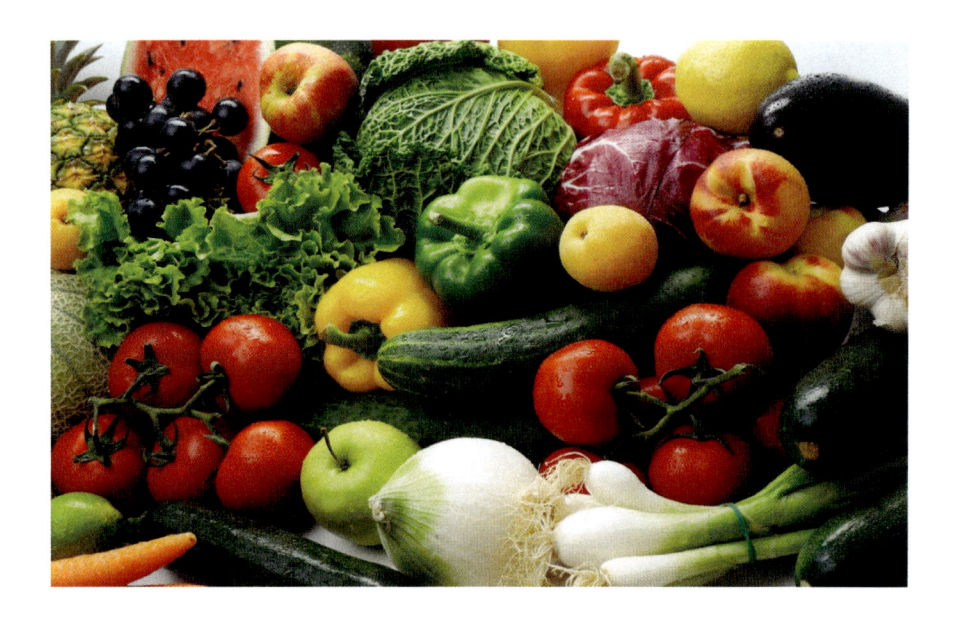

Whether you choose to eat the Paleo diet or not, the following key factors apply to any "healthy diet":

1. Eliminate all gluten
2. Eliminate all artificial sweeteners, especially aspartame
3. Do eat unprocessed whole foods
4. Do eat organic or grass fed foods that are free from additives and genetically modified ingredients.
5. Carbohydrates should primarily come from vegetables (except corn and potatoes, which should typically be avoided.) Dramatically lowering your intake of non-vegetable carbohydrates could improve insulin signaling, which can also improve migraines.

Another factor related to diet and sometimes overlooked is the existence of food allergies. Besides being aware of any foods that trigger a headache after you eat them, additional questions that can help you determine if you have a food allergy include:

1. Do you experience bloating after eating certain foods?
2. Do you have constipation/diarrhea after eating certain foods?
3. Do certain foods give you a stuffy nose, wheezing or shortness of breath?
4. Do you have low energy or feel drowsy after eating certain foods?

If you answered yes to any of these questions, you may want to keep a detailed food journal to start tracking potential migraine-inducing foods. Keep in mind that eliminating your migraines is not the only health benefit you can reap from identifying food allergies or sensitivities. Eliminating food antigens is also critical for gut health, which leads to overall health.

In a 1979 study published in "Lancet", sixty migraine sufferers with food antigen immunoreactivity who were put on an elimination diet experienced profound relief. According to the author, "the commonest foods causing reactions were: wheat 78%, oranges 65%, non-organic eggs 45%, tea and coffee 40% each, chocolate and milk 37% each, non-organic beef 35% and corn, cane sugar and yeast 33% each." When an average of 10 common foods were avoided, there was a dramatic fall in the numbers of headaches per month. 85 percent of patients became headache free.[xiv]

Nutritional Supplements for Headache Relief

There are several nutritional supplements that can help reduce and prevent headaches and migraines. Some of the best ones include:

CO Q10

In terms of supplements that might be helpful for the treatment of migraines, one of the most critical is ubiquenol (the reduced form of Q10). According to experts, an underlying problem involved with migraines is mitochondrial dysfunction. Ubiquenol plays a vital role in ATP production, which is the basic fuel for your mitochondria. Our bodies do produce ubiquenol naturally; in fact it is the predominant form in most healthy cells, tissues and organs. However, with rampant pollution and poor diet, mitochondrial dysfunction has become increasingly common.

A 2005 study published in "Neurology" found that CO Q10 was superior to a placebo in preventing migraines and reducing severity. Of the patients that received 100 mg of CO Q10 three times a day, 50% reported significantly reduced frequency of headaches compared to only 14% of those who took the placebo. Ubiquenol is the reduced form of CO Q10 and studies have repeatedly demonstrated that it is far more effective than CO Q10 due to its superior bioavailability.[xv]

Magnesium

Magnesium is probably the most important supplement for headaches and migraines, since it serves to relax the blood vessels that cause the pain. The best magnesium supplement is Magnesium Threonate because it penetrates all membranes, including the mitochondria, and no other magnesium supplement does this. 600 mg to 800 mg a day is recommended. Interestingly, some of the best drugs used to treat migraines are calcium blockers, and that is how magnesium works. Supplemental magnesium would be far safer than taking a calcium channel blocker.

Butterbur Root

Another natural supplement that has been shown to reduce migraine symptoms is something called Butterbur Root. Butterbur (petasites hybridus) is a plant that has been used since ancient times for a wide range of medicinal purposes in Europe. Butterbur extracts possess analgesic, anti-inflammatory, anti-spasmodic and vasodilatatory properties, which explains its efficiency in treating migraines. Butterbur root extract (standardized to 15% petasins) has been shown to be both safe and effective for the prevention of migraines.[xvi]

In one study, researchers split 245 patients into three groups to receive 75 mg of butterbur root extract twice a day, or 50 mg of butterbur extract twice a day or a placebo. At the end of the four-month treatment period, those taking the 75 mg dosage experienced a dramatic 48% reduction in the frequency of the migraine attacks.[xvii]

Butterbur is so effective at reducing the frequency and severity of migraine attacks that the American Academy of Neurology (AAN) and American Headache Society (AHS) have both recommended this supplement as an effective treatment for migraines.[xviii]

Riboflavin

Riboflavin (B2) is another promising supplement for migraine relief. Vitamin B2 contributes to cell growth, enzyme function and energy production.[xix] It is believed that riboflavin's beneficial effects are due to its ability to enhance mitochondrial energy production.[xx] This is based on data indicating that riboflavin is especially effective among migraine patients with mitochondrial genetic abnormalities.[xxi] One study involving 23 participants showed that taking 400 mg of riboflavin supplements daily-reduced headache frequency by an impressive 50% in 3 months.[xxii]

Melatonin

Melatonin is another very effective treatment for migraines. It is a natural compound produced by the pineal gland that helps regulate sleep-wake cycles (circadian rhythms) and has been shown to have potent antioxidant and analgesic properties. Since melatonin is often found in the lower than normal levels among migraine sufferers, especially during an attack, some researchers hypothesize that migraines are triggered by an irregularity in pineal gland function. [xxiii]

In one study, melatonin supplementation showed a two-thirds reduction in the number of migraine attacks.[xxiv] This response rate may have been more statistically significant if the researchers used a larger dose (3 mg instead of 2mg) and an increase in treatment time (12-16 weeks instead of 8 weeks).

Adenosylmelhionine and L-Tryptophan

Low serotonin levels have been another clinically significant finding in migraine sufferers. Two supplements known to increase serotonin are S. Adenosylmelhionine, otherwise known as Sam E (400 – 800 mg recommended daily) and L-Tryptophan, an amino acid that is a precursor to serotonin.[xxv]

The fact that these supplements help ease migraines is evidence that low serotonergic signaling within the brain may precipitate a migraine. Therefore, supporting serotonin synthesis by providing precursors like L-Tryptophan may help avoid physiological conditions that promote a migraine headache. In an older clinical trial, supplementation with 2-4 grams of L-Tryptophan daily was as effective at preventing migraine attacks as the medication methysergide. A more recent study found that dietary tryptophan depletion caused an exacerbation of migraine symptoms.[xxvi]

As you can see, preventing neck pain and headaches can be a multi-faceted approach as there is more than one cause as to why people suffer from headaches. That's why a comprehensive approach is the best way to get rid of your headaches in the next 30 days:

1. Get a thorough muscle palpation exam, including x-rays of the cervical spine and a MRI of the cervical spine and brain before any treatment is administered.
2. Take inventory of any past accidents or injuries.
3. Evaluate past and current physical ergonomics, being sure to correct forward head posture as much as possible. Remember, 90 percent of all headaches are muscle contraction/tension headaches and are related to subluxation and poor posture.
4. Take supplements, including L-Tryptophan (2-4 grams per day), Riboflavin (400 mg per day), Sam E (400-800 mg per day), Melatonin (3 mg per day), Butterbur (75 mg 2x per day), Magnesium (800 mg per day), and CQ 10 (100 mg 3x per day).
5. Eliminate gluten and all artificial sweeteners, especially aspartame, flavorings like

MSG, and preservatives like the nitrates that are found in most processed meats.
6. Avoid foods with tryamine, such as processed meats, canned foods, aged cheese and red wine.
7. Consider eating a Paleo Diet, that consists of only non processed foods.
8. Engage in healthy exercises, such as walking, swimming or yoga to reduce stress.

A well rounded approach "leaves no stone unturned" and will give you the very best chance of living a healthy, headache-free life. Take the steps you need to put yourself in charge of your health. You no longer have to play victim to your headaches. You can step into the driver's seat and kiss your head pain good-bye.

Personal Case Studies

Case Study 1

Some years ago, a mother came into my office to inquire if I treated headaches. She told me that they lived in the neighborhood and passed by my office quite frequently. She explained that her 15-year old daughter had been suffering from such severe headaches that she stopped going to school. Her mother explained that she started these headaches about 2 years ago and had been seen by numerous doctors, including a special headache clinic in Chicago. No one was able to figure out the cause or any real solution. The daughter was finally seen by a psychiatrist and diagnosed as manic-depressive and put on lithium, along with other medications.

A couple days later, she brought her daughter, whom I'll call Mary, in to see me. I found her to be a well adjusted young girl despite the fact that she had been confined to her bed between 16-18 hours per day due to a combination of headaches and the side effects of the medications she was taking. The final diagnosis for Mary was that there was no real reason that she should be suffering from these headaches, that she was manifesting her headaches as a part of a manic depressive syndrome. That was when the lithium was prescribed and Mary's life had come to an end. You can understand her parent's frustration and desperation at this point.

Upon speaking with Mary, I asked her about when her headaches began and if there was anything of significance that had occurred in her life around that time. Mary said that she was a passenger in a motor vehicle accident about 6 months prior and that was the only thing she could think of. I asked where the headaches seem to come from and she explained that they seem to originate at the back of her neck just below her skull and then come across into her temple and over her eye, usually one side or the other. Mary stated that she had been voicing this to the other specialists, but was told that the neck had nothing to do with the head and that it was not the problem.

After palpating the muscles and vertebrae at the top of Mary's neck, I found a severe subluxation, or misalignment, at the top two vertebrae C1-C2. That was good news because there was a direct connection from where Mary's pain began and the cause of her headaches. Next, a front and side view x-ray was taken, which confirmed my belief. Mary's C2 vertebra was rotated severely, causing pressure on the vertebral arteries and vascular changes into the back of her head.

I began treating Mary with chiropractic adjustments, along with sub occipital soft tissue technique and a special type of lordotic traction. Mary also had a reversal of the normal cervical curve, Forward Head Posture, adding to the stress and tension of her head.

After four weeks of intense treatment at 3 times per week, Mary was able to cut her medication in half and her headaches reduced from daily to 1 to 2 times per week. After another 4 weeks of treatment at 2 times per week, Mary was completely off all her medications and for the first time in 2 years, she experienced a full week with no medication and no headaches.

Since that time, Mary has sought treatment 1-2 times per month just for maintenance care and has remained headache free.

After the first month, her parents were ecstatic. They couldn't believe there was such a simple solution to this up until now undiagnosed disability. They couldn't believe the look in their daughter's eyes, happy, cheerful and alive, a look that they hadn't seen in two years, a look that they had worried they may never see again. Finally, they had their daughter back!!

The reaction over the next couple of weeks was interesting. The parents began to realize what would have happened if it weren't for a chance meeting (I believe it was meant to be!). No doctor ever even suggested going to a chiropractor. Not one doctor asked about the car accident, let alone connected the dots, and they had been to specialists around the country. The next reaction was anger. They could not believe what almost happened. You can imagine what they felt. But the important thing is that Mary has her life back and that's all that matters!

Case Study 2

Some years later, I was confronted with a very unusual and probably the most challenging situation in my career. A mother brought in her 18 year old son to me, whom I'll call Peter. He had been involved in a motor vehicle accident about two years before. The accident was very severe; his car had slid off the road into a telephone pole at about 40-50 mph. His car didn't have air bags and his seat belt had failed. Peter was sent through the front windshield at a very high velocity. He had fractured five out of seven cervical vertebrae. There were two surgeries performed; one going through the back of the neck, and another across the front of his throat. Five out of the seven vertebrae were fused with screws and bolts.

Peter had recovered fully from the surgeries, but was left with severe migraines that had become a chronic daily event. Peter also had severe restriction of movement, which could easily be understood, along with a throbbing pressure at the base of the neck, which shot into both temples around his eyes. Due to the severity of the surgery, the orthopedic doctors told his mother that no chiropractic or physical therapy should ever be done to his neck.

Peter's mother had brought him into me against doctor's orders just to see if anything could be done. She knew her son couldn't live the rest of his life this way, but no one had any solutions.

After a cervical x-ray, I found something very interesting - Peter's neck had been fused in perfect alignment from C3 to C7, but the first two vertebrae, C1 and C2 were rotated in the opposite direction.

In the doctor's rush to save Peter's life and stabilize his cervical spine, the top two vertebrae, which were not fractured, were omitted from surgical intervention. Due to the severity of the accident, the head trauma and neck injury, the orthopedic surgeons had their hands full. The challenge was to fix Peter's top two vertebrae without putting any stress on the rest of the cervical spine. Most orthopedics don't realize that a chiropractic adjustment in experienced hands can be very specific.

At first, myofascial work was done on the upper cervical spine, the sternocleidomastoid muscle (SCM) and both trapezius muscles. Passive stretching was then gently applied and after a week, Peter received his first chiropractic adjustment at C1-C2. Over the next couple of weeks, Peter began to notice a dramatic decrease in the frequency and severity of his headaches. And unexpectedly, there was also an increase in his range of motion. At the six-week mark, Peter had his first full week with no medication and no headaches. After another two weeks, a follow-up x-ray was taken, which showed a full correction at the C1-C2 vertebral level. Peter has come in periodically for a maintenance check-up, but remains headache free to this day.

Case Study 3

This is a unique situation because Jarred is my son. When Jarred was four years old, he had three neck and head injuries within 6 months. One of the last injuries actually sent him to the hospital with a concussion. A couple of months after his last injury, Jarred started complaining of headaches.

Initially, he had an MRI of the brain to rule out any internal bleeding. After that test came back negative, I did an evaluation, which included muscle palpation and a cervical x-ray. My son, at the age of four, was showing a C2 spinous rotation (misalignment). He also had tenderness at the top of the neck and joint fixation at that level.

Jarred received his first adjustment at four years old. I adjusted him twice a week for a month. After that, I adjusted him once a week for another month. After the first month, he told me his headaches were gone. Today my son is 17 years old and I usually adjust him once a month to keep him headache free.

I do believe that he suffered some ligament damage because his neck is still a weak area. But with periodic maintenance care, he remains headache free. The interesting fact is that he does not remember any of the accidents that occurred at age four. I wonder how many of us forget injuries that occurred to us over the years that play a major role in what is happening to us today.

FAQ's

Does the spine have anything to do with my headaches?

Absolutely, especially the upper parts of the neck, the first two vertebrae near the back of the head. C1-C2 controls the blood supply, along with cerebral spine fluid (CSF) in and out of the brain.

Why are my headaches worse when the weather gets rainy?

Atmospheric pressure can affect the sinuses, and in some people, it can cause sinus pressure. Increased swelling will create a sinus type headache, usually over the temples and around the eyes. In a recent survey by the National Headache Foundation, patients were given a list of 16 triggers. Three out of every four respondents said that weather triggered their headache pain.

Specific weather triggers include:

- Changes in humidity
- Changes in temperature
- Storms
- Extremely dry conditions
- Dusty environments

How long will I have to undergo treatment to find any relief?

It depends on how long you have been suffering. Usually, with any condition, the longer the problem has existed, the longer the treatment to correct it may take. Typically though, most people will find significant relief within 30 days of chiropractic treatment, along with ergonomic and dietary changes.

Why doesn't the medication I take always work?

Again, each person is different. What works for one person may not work for another. Also, if your headaches are primarily muscle tension/migraine headaches, which are the most common, just taking a pill does not solve the problem. If there is a misalignment at the top of the neck causing restricted blood flow due to tension on the vertebral arteries, medication will only give very temporary relief at best.

How will the chiropractic adjustments work if my headaches are sinus related?

There are many causes of headaches, but some people are particularly sensitive to sinus headaches. Chiropractic care works extremely well in relieving sinus type headaches due to a combination of soft tissue mobilization techniques to the base of the skull at the top of the neck, along with acupressure massage on the temple and forehead above the eyes, and in front of the cheek bones. These are the sinus pressure points, and it is very effective in relieving sinus headaches. Many times, I will include peppermint and eucalyptus so the patient can inhale these while I administer the acupressure massage. Nutritional supplements called bromelain and quercetin are also helpful in relieving sinus pain because they reduce inflammation.

Should I take medication in conjunction with chiropractic adjustments?

There is nothing wrong with taking medication on a short-term basis as long as treatment is focused on looking for and correcting the cause of the problem. The goal is to help the person rely less and less on medication.

Will I have to continue chiropractic treatment for the rest of my life?

The best answer to this question depends on the individual and the amount of the spinal injury that has been caused. Some people require only a short amount of chiropractic care to be healed. Other people who have had a long-term condition or multiple injuries, such as multiple car accidents, will require some supplemental care that may be ongoing. Either way, a good analogy would be comparing chiropractic care to dentistry. After a problem has been corrected, ongoing dental checkups 1-2 times per year is recommended to maintain good dental health. The same is true with spinal check-ups. The final decision is of course always up to each individual.

Are there any therapies I can do at home to help alleviate my headaches other than medication?

Some of the most natural remedies other than prescription medication are as follows:

Magnesium (800 mg per day)
- Butterbur Root (75 mg 2x per day)
- L-tryptophan (4 g per day)
- Melatonin (3 mg per day)
- Sam E (600 mg per day)
- Riboflavin (600 mg per day)

Also, remember to avoid forward head posture:

- Avoid sleeping on the couch with pillows behind the neck. Avoid reading in bed.

Adjust all computer screens to eye level.

APPENDIX A

Further Information on the Deleterious Effect of NSAiDs

While inhibition of Cox1 can have serious gastro-intestinal consequences, selective inhibition of Cox2 carries cardiovascular risks. Blood platelets express thromboxane A2 (TXA2), a blood clotting, vessel-constricting compound that is synthesized by Cox1. Blood vessels produce an anti-clotting compound called prostaglandin 12 (PG12). During a blood vessel injury, the relative ratios of TXA2 and PG12 are controlled by Cox enzymes to balance the opposing action of clotting and blood flow. Cox2 specific inhibitors (e.g. coxibs) preferentially reduce amounts of PG12, tipping the balance toward thrombosis.[xxvii] The increased risk of thrombosis and heart attack observed in some studies of Cox2 inhibitors may result from this mechanism.[xxviii]

Increase in blood vessel constriction by Cox2 inhibition can also lead to the hypertension and renal failure seen in some studies of non-selective and Cox2 selective NSAids. Cox2 inhibitors may also impair the removal of excess cholesterol from the blood vessel walls, a process known as reverse cholesterol transport.[xxix]

An underappreciated side effect of NSAiD use is kidney toxicity. Long-term use of NSAiDs can lead to impaired glomerular filtration, renal tubular necrosis, and ultimately, chronic renal failure by disrupting prostaglandin synthesis, which can impair renal blood flow.[xxx] This is because prostaglandins, which are blocked by cox inhibition, are important for proper blood vessel function within the kidneys.[xxxi]

NSAiDs can also contribute to mitochondrial dysfunction, causing the formation of highly reactive free radicals, which cause tissue damage and may contribute to toxicity associated with NSAiDs.[xxxii] As I stated earlier, mitochondrial dysfunction has been linked to the development of migraines in a 2005 study published in *Neurology*. The study also shows that COQ10 acts as a basic fuel to the mitochondrial, helping to prevent and reduce the intensity of a migraine. When the mitochondria are functioning normally, they generate minimal oxidative products and the body's antioxidant defense systems keep them in check. However, when toxins, in this case, NSAiDs or their metabolites, interfere with the efficiency of this process, the amount of free radicals generated is increased considerably.[xxxiii] This mechanism has been shown to cause gastrointestinal and liver toxicity.[xxxiv]

[i] http://www.healthline.com/health/mixed-tension-migraine#Overview%201

[ii] http://www.who.int/mediacentre/factsheets/fs277/en/

[iii] http://www.health.harvard.edu/healthbeat/what-type-of-headache-do-you-have

[iv] Kapandji, I. A. (2008) *The Physiology of the Joints, volume III.* Retrieved from http://books.google.com/books/about/The_physiology_of_the_joints.html?id=k5wTAQAAMAAJ

[v]
http://www.health.harvard.edu/press_releases/acetaminophen_overdose

[vi] *Acetaminophen and NSAID Toxicity.* Life Extension. http://www.lef.org/PDFMaker/MakePDF.aspx?a=1&pdf=1&fn=LE-PAGEID-113717&url=http://www.lef.org/Health-Well-

ness/LECMS/PrintVersionMagic.aspx?CmsID=113717

[vii] *Acetaminophen and NSAID Toxicity.* Life Extension. http://www.lef.org/PDFMaker/MakePDF.aspx?a=1&pdf=1&fn=LE-PAGEID-113717&url=http://www.lef.org/Health-Well-ness/LECMS/PrintVersionMagic.aspx?CmsID=113717

[viii]

http://www.health.harvard.edu/press_releases/acetaminophen_overdose

[ix] *Acetaminophen and NSAID Toxicity.* Life Extension. http://www.lef.org/PDFMaker/MakePDF.aspx?a=1&pdf=1&fn=LE-PAGEID-113717&url=http://www.lef.org/Health-Well-ness/LECMS/PrintVersionMagic.aspx?CmsID=113717

[x] *Acetaminophen and NSAID Toxicity.* Life Extension. http://www.lef.org/PDFMaker/MakePDF.aspx?a=1&pdf=1&fn=LE-PAGEID-113717&url=http://www.lef.org/Health-Well-

ness/LECMS/PrintVersionMagic.aspx?CmsID=113717

[xi] *Acetaminophen and NSAID Toxicity.* Life Extension. http://www.lef.org/PDFMaker/MakePDF.aspx?a=1&pdf=1&fn=LE-PAGEID-113717&url=http://www.lef.org/Health-Well-ness/LECMS/PrintVersionMagic.aspx?CmsID=113717

[xii] *Acetaminophen and NSAID Toxicity.* Life Extension. http://www.lef.org/PDFMaker/MakePDF.aspx?a=1&pdf=1&fn=LE-PAGEID-113717&url=http://www.lef.org/Health-Well-ness/LECMS/PrintVersionMagic.aspx?CmsID=113717

[xiii] http://www.mayoclinic.org/healthy-living/stress-management/in-depth/yoga/art-20044733

[xiv] Lancet 1979 May 5;1(8123):966-9 http://www.ncbi.nlm.nih.gov/pubmed/87628

[xv] Neurology 2005 Aug 23;65(4):580-5
http://www.ncbi.nlm.nih.gov/pubmed/16116119

[xvi] Pothmann, R; Danesch, U. *Migraine Prevention in Children and Adolescents: Results of an Open Study With a Special Butterbur Root Extract.* http://www.google.com/url?sa=t&rct=j&q=&esrc=s&source=web&cd=2&ved=0CC4QFjAB&url=http%3A%2F%2Fwww.petasites.eu%2FPDF%2FPoth-mann_Headache.pdf&ei=bEbQU5D6L86wyASOr4GQAg&usg=AFQjCNFJNcr-Ki-wIpXtHRLSD5WkJhRr5Jw&sig2=Gyfbc9g_luqzM2b52_TS1Q&bvm=bv.71667212,d.aWw

[xvii] Lipton, R. B. Neurology 2004 Dec 28;63(12):2240-4
http://www.ncbi.nlm.nih.gov/pubmed/15623680

[xviii] Holland, S. Neurology April 24, 2012 vol. 78 no. 17 1346-1353
http://www.neurology.org/content/78/17/1346.full

[xix] Alternative Medicine Review Volume 13, Number 4 2008. Riboflavin. Thorne Research http://www.thorne.com/altmedrev/.fulltext/13/4/334.pdf

[xx] http://www.lef.org/protocols/health_concerns/migraine_07.htm

[xxi] DiLorenzo, C. Neurology. 2009 May 5;72(18):1588-94 http://www.ncbi.nlm.nih.gov/pubmed/19414726

[xxii] Boehnke, C. Eur J Neurol. 2004 Jul;11(7):475-7. http://www.ncbi.nlm.nih.gov/pubmed/15257686

[xxiii] http://www.lef.org/protocols/health_concerns/migraine_07.htm

[xxiv] Alstadhaug, K. B. Neurology. 2010 Oct 26;75(17):1527-32.

http://www.ncbi.nlm.nih.gov/pubmed/20975054

[xxv] http://www.lef.org/protocols/health_concerns/migraine_07.htm

[xxvi] Drummond, P. D. Cephalalgia. 2006 Oct;26(10):1225-33.
http://www.ncbi.nlm.nih.gov/pubmed/16961791

[xxvii] Vonkemen, H. E. Eur J Clin Pharmacol. 2013 Mar;69(3):365-71.
http://www.ncbi.nlm.nih.gov/pubmed/22890587

[xxviii] Conaghan, P. G. Rheumatol Int. 2012 Jun;32(6):1491-502
http://www.ncbi.nlm.nih.gov/pubmed/22193214

[xxix] http://orthoinfo.aaos.org/topic.cfm?topic=A00284&webid=23DBE45E

[xxx] Weir, M. R. Cleve Clin J Med. 2002;69 Suppl 1:SI53-8. http://www.ncbi.nlm.nih.gov/pubmed/12086295

[xxxi] Ejaz, P. J Assoc Physicians India. 2004 Aug;52:632-40. http://www.ncbi.nlm.nih.gov/pubmed/15847359

[xxxii]

http://www.lef.org/protocols/appendix/otc_toxicity_03.htm

[xxxiii]

http://www.lef.org/protocols/appendix/otc_toxicity_03.htm

[xxxiv] Watanabe, T. J Clin Biochem Nutr. Mar 2011; 48(2): 117–121.

http://www.ncbi.nlm.nih.gov/pmc/articles/PMC3045683/

Made in the USA
Monee, IL
26 August 2020